DR ALMEDA J. BIERMAN

Intermittent Fasting for Weight Loss and Wellness

A Beginner's Guide to Losing fat, Feeling More Energized, and Boosting Your Health with Fasting

Contents

About the Author

Dr. Almeda J. Bierman is an expert in the field of nutrition and wellness. With a passion for helping others achieve optimal health, Dr. Bierman has dedicated her career to researching and educating individuals on the benefits of a balanced and mindful approach to eating.

As a highly respected doctor, Dr. Bierman has spent years studying the intricate relationship between food, metabolism, and overall well-being.

Dr. Bierman's approach to intermittent fasting is rooted in scientific research and evidence-based practices. She believes in the power of intermittent fasting as a tool for weight management, improving metabolic health, and promoting overall wellness.

In addition to her academic achievements, Dr. Bierman is a dedicated advocate for a holistic approach to health. She believes that true well-being encompasses not only physical health but also mental and emotional well-being. Her holistic perspective shines through in her writing, as she encourages readers to embrace a balanced lifestyle that nourishes both the body and the soul.

When she's not immersed in her research or writing, Dr. Bierman enjoys spending time in nature, practicing mindfulness, and exploring new recipes in her kitchen. She believes in leading by example and incorporates the principles of intermittent fasting into her own life, experiencing firsthand the positive impact it can have on overall well-being.

Introduction

Welcome to the world of intermittent fasting, where you can achieve your weight loss and wellness goals while enjoying a flexible and sustainable approach to eating. If you've ever struggled with traditional diets or felt overwhelmed by complicated meal plans, then this book is for you.

As someone who has personally experienced the transformative power of intermittent fasting, I am excited to share with you the knowledge and insights that will help you embark on this incredible journey towards a healthier and happier version of yourself.

But before we dive into the details, let me assure you that intermittent fasting is not just another fad diet. It is a scientifically-backed and time-tested method that has been practiced for centuries. It taps into the natural rhythms of our bodies and allows us to harness the incredible potential within us to achieve sustainable weight loss and overall wellness.

In this book, we will explore the basics of intermittent fasting, understand how it works, and uncover the numerous benefits it offers. We will discuss different methods of intermittent fasting and help you choose the one that best suits your lifestyle and goals.

But this book is not just about the "what" and the "how" of intermittent fasting. It's about empowering you with the knowledge and tools to make informed decisions about your health. We will address common myths and misconceptions surrounding intermittent fasting, ensuring that you have a clear understanding of what to expect and what not to believe.

Throughout this journey, I will be your guide, providing practical tips and strategies to make your intermittent fasting experience a success. From managing hunger and cravings to incorporating exercise, I will share with you the secrets to staying on track and achieving optimal results.

But don't just take my word for it. This book is also enriched with real-life success stories from individuals who have embraced intermittent fasting and witnessed remarkable transformations in their lives. Their stories will inspire and motivate you, proving that you too can achieve your weight loss and wellness goals with the power of intermittent fasting.

So, are you ready to unlock the secrets to a healthier you? Are you ready to say goodbye to restrictive diets and hello to a sustainable lifestyle? If so, let's embark on this journey together and discover the incredible benefits that intermittent fasting can bring to your life.

Remember, this is not just a book; it's a roadmap to a better version of yourself. Let's dive in and embrace the power of intermittent fasting for weight loss and wellness!

Understanding the Basics of Intermittent Fasting

In order to fully grasp the concept of intermittent fasting, it's essential to understand what it is and how it works. So, let's dive into the basics and unravel the secrets behind this powerful approach to eating.

What is Intermittent Fasting?

Intermittent fasting is not a diet in the traditional sense. It's an eating pattern that cycles between periods of fasting and eating. Unlike most diets that focus on what you eat, intermittent fasting is more concerned with when you eat.

The concept is simple: you alternate between periods of eating and fasting. During the fasting period, you abstain from consuming calories, allowing your body to tap into its fat stores for energy. The eating period, also known as the "feeding window," is when you consume your meals.

How Does Intermittent Fasting Work?

Intermittent fasting works by tapping into the body's natural metabolic processes. When you fast, your body undergoes several changes that can have profound effects on your health and weight.

One of the key mechanisms behind intermittent fasting is insulin regulation. When you eat, your body releases insulin to help transport glucose from the bloodstream into the cells for energy. However, constant eating throughout the day can lead to chronically elevated insulin levels, which can promote weight gain and other health issues.

By incorporating periods of fasting, you give your body a break from constantly producing insulin. This allows insulin levels to normalize, leading to improved insulin sensitivity. When your body becomes more sensitive to insulin, it can more effectively regulate blood sugar levels and promote fat burning.

Additionally, during fasting periods, your body enters a state called ketosis. Ketosis occurs when your body switches from using glucose as its primary fuel source to using stored fat for energy. This can lead to significant fat loss and improved body composition.

Different Methods of Intermittent Fasting

There are several different methods of intermittent fasting, allowing you to choose the one that best fits your lifestyle and preferences. Here are some popular approaches:

1. 16/8 Method: This method involves fasting for 16 hours and restricting your eating window to 8 hours. For example, you

may choose to eat between 12 pm and 8 pm, and then fast until the next day at noon.

2. 5:2 Diet: With this method, you eat normally for five days of the week and restrict your calorie intake to 500-600 calories for two non-consecutive days. These fasting days should not be consecutive to allow for adequate nourishment.

3. Alternate-Day Fasting: As the name suggests, this method involves alternating between fasting days and regular eating days. On fasting days, you consume little to no calories, while on eating days, you eat normally.

4. Eat-Stop-Eat: This method involves fasting for 24 hours once or twice a week. For example, you may choose to fast from dinner one day until dinner the next day.

5. Warrior Diet: This method involves fasting during the day and having one large meal at night. During the fasting period, you can consume small amounts of raw fruits and vegetables, as well as fluids like water and herbal tea.

It's important to note that while intermittent fasting can be highly effective, it may not be suitable for everyone. It's always recommended to consult with a healthcare professional before starting any new dietary regimen, especially if you have underlying health conditions or are taking medications.

Understanding the basics of intermittent fasting sets the foundation for your journey towards weight loss and wellness. In the next section, we will explore the incredible benefits that intermittent fasting can offer, from shedding excess pounds to improving overall health and well-being.

Benefits of Intermittent Fasting

Intermittent fasting not only offers a unique approach to weight loss but also provides a wide range of benefits for your overall health and well-being. Let's explore some of the incredible advantages that intermittent fasting can bring to your life.

Weight Loss

One of the primary reasons why people turn to intermittent fasting is its effectiveness in promoting weight loss. By incorporating periods of fasting, you create a calorie deficit, which is essential for shedding excess pounds. Additionally, intermittent fasting can help boost your metabolism, increase fat burning, and reduce overall calorie intake.

Improved Insulin Sensitivity

Insulin sensitivity refers to how well your body responds to insulin, the hormone responsible for regulating blood sugar levels. Poor insulin sensitivity can lead to weight gain, type 2 diabetes, and other metabolic disorders. Intermittent fasting has been shown to improve insulin sensitivity, allowing your body to better control blood sugar levels and potentially reduce the risk of developing insulin resistance.

Enhanced Brain Function

Intermittent fasting has been linked to improved brain health and cognitive function. During fasting periods, your body undergoes cellular repair processes, including the removal of waste materials and the production of new cells. This process, known as autophagy, can help protect against neurodegenerative diseases and improve overall brain function.

Increased Autophagy

Autophagy, as mentioned earlier, is the body's natural process of cellular repair and regeneration. During fasting, autophagy is upregulated, leading to the removal of damaged cells and the recycling of cellular components. This process can help slow down the aging process, improve cellular health, and reduce the risk of chronic diseases.

Reduced Inflammation

Chronic inflammation is a common underlying factor in many health conditions, including obesity, heart disease, and certain types of cancer. Intermittent fasting has been shown to reduce inflammation markers in the body, potentially lowering the risk of developing inflammatory diseases and improving overall health.

Longevity and Anti-Aging

Research suggests that intermittent fasting may have anti-aging effects and promote longevity. By reducing oxidative stress, improving cellular repair mechanisms, and enhancing metabolic flexibility, intermittent fasting can potentially slow down the aging process and increase lifespan.

These are just a few of the many benefits that intermittent fasting can offer. It's important to note that individual results may vary, and the extent of these benefits depends on various factors such as lifestyle, diet, and overall health.

Now that you understand the incredible advantages of intermittent fasting, it's time to dive deeper into the practical aspects. In the next section, we will discuss how to get started with intermittent fasting, including important considerations and steps to ensure a successful journey.

Getting Started with Intermittent Fasting

Consultation with a Healthcare Professional

Before embarking on any new dietary regimen, including intermittent fasting, it is crucial to consult with a healthcare professional. While intermittent fasting can offer numerous benefits, it may not be suitable for everyone, especially those with certain medical conditions or individuals who are taking specific medications. Let's explore why seeking professional guidance is essential and what you can expect during a consultation.

Why Consult with a Healthcare Professional?

1. Personalized Advice: A healthcare professional can provide personalized advice based on your unique health history, current medications, and any underlying medical conditions. They can assess whether intermittent fasting is safe and appropriate for you, taking into account any potential risks or contraindications.

2. Monitoring of Health Markers: Certain medical conditions, such as diabetes or hormonal imbalances, may require careful monitoring while practicing intermittent fasting. A healthcare professional can help track your health markers, such as blood sugar levels, cholesterol levels, and hormone levels, to ensure that intermittent fasting does not negatively impact your health.

3. Optimal Nutrition: While intermittent fasting focuses on when you eat rather than what you eat, it's still essential to maintain a balanced and nutritious diet during your eating periods. A healthcare professional can provide guidance on how to structure your meals to ensure you are meeting your nutritional needs and getting all the essential vitamins and minerals.

4. Medication Adjustments: If you are taking medications, intermittent fasting may affect their absorption or metabolism. A healthcare professional can evaluate your medication regimen and make any necessary adjustments to ensure their effectiveness and safety while practicing intermittent fasting.

What to Expect During a Consultation?

When you schedule a consultation with a healthcare professional, here's what you can expect:

1. Medical History Review: The healthcare professional will review your medical history, including any existing conditions, past surgeries, and current medications. It's important to provide accurate and detailed information to ensure a comprehensive evaluation.

2. Discussion of Goals: You will have the opportunity to discuss your goals for practicing intermittent fasting, whether it's weight loss, improved metabolic health, or other specific objectives. This will help the healthcare professional tailor their advice to align with your goals.

3. Physical Examination: In some cases, a physical examination may be conducted to assess your overall health status. This may include measurements such as blood pressure, body weight, and body composition analysis.

4. Blood Tests: Depending on your medical history and specific concerns, the healthcare professional may recommend blood tests to assess your baseline health markers. These tests can provide valuable insights into your metabolic health and help monitor any changes during intermittent fasting.

5. Guidance and Recommendations: Based on the information gathered, the healthcare professional will provide guidance and recommendations tailored to your needs. This may include specific intermittent fasting protocols, meal planning advice, and lifestyle modifications to support your overall well-being.

Remember, the consultation with a healthcare professional is an opportunity to gain valuable insights and ensure that intermittent fasting is safe and suitable for you. Their expertise and guidance can help you navigate the journey with confidence and optimize your results.

Choosing the Right Intermittent Fasting Method

When it comes to intermittent fasting, there are several different methods to choose from. Each method has its own unique approach and fasting window duration. It's important to select the right intermittent fasting method that aligns with your lifestyle, preferences, and health goals. In this section, we will explore some popular intermittent fasting methods to help you make an informed decision.

1. 16/8 Method (Leangains Protocol)

The 16/8 method, also known as the Leangains Protocol, involves fasting for 16 hours and restricting your eating window to 8 hours each day. This method is popular because it can be easily incorporated into daily routines. For example, you might choose to skip breakfast and have your first meal at noon, followed by your last meal at 8 pm. During the fasting period, you can consume calorie-free beverages like water, black coffee, or herbal tea.

2. 5:2 Diet

The 5:2 diet involves eating normally for five days of the week and restricting calorie intake to 500-600 calories for the remaining two days. On fasting days, it's important to choose nutrient-dense foods to ensure you're getting essential vitamins and minerals despite the reduced calorie intake. This method provides flexibility, as you can choose which days to fast based on your schedule and preferences.

3. Alternate-Day Fasting

Alternate-day fasting involves alternating between fasting days and regular eating days. On fasting days, you consume little to no calories, while on eating days, you can eat normally. This method can be more challenging for some individuals, as it involves full-day fasting. However, it can be effective for weight loss and improving insulin sensitivity.

4. Eat-Stop-Eat

The Eat-Stop-Eat method involves fasting for 24 hours once or twice a week. For example, you might choose to fast from dinner one day until dinner the next day. During the fasting period, only calorie-free beverages are allowed. This method may require more discipline and planning, but it can provide significant benefits, including weight loss and improved cellular repair.

5. Warrior Diet

The Warrior Diet follows a 20-hour fasting period, followed by a 4-hour eating window. During the fasting period, small amounts of raw fruits and vegetables, as well as protein-rich foods, are allowed. The main meal is consumed during the 4-hour eating window, typically in the evening. This method is inspired by ancient warrior cultures and aims to align with our natural circadian rhythms.

Considerations for Choosing the Right Method

When choosing the right intermittent fasting method for you, consider the following factors:

1. Lifestyle: Select a method that fits seamlessly into your daily routine and lifestyle. Consider your work schedule, social commitments, and personal preferences.

2. Health Goals: Determine your specific health goals, whether it's weight loss, improved metabolic health, or increased energy levels. Different methods may have varying effects on these goals.

3. Sustainability: Choose a method that you can sustain in the long term. It's important to find an intermittent fasting approach that you can comfortably incorporate into your lifestyle without feeling deprived or overwhelmed.

4. Individual Needs: Consider any individual needs or health conditions you may have. If you have a medical condition or take medications, consult with a healthcare professional to ensure the chosen method is safe and suitable for you.

Setting Realistic Goals

Setting realistic goals is an essential component of any successful endeavor, and this holds true for intermittent fasting as well. When embarking on an intermittent fasting journey, it's important to establish goals that are both achievable and sustainable. In this section, we will explore the importance of setting realistic goals and provide practical tips to help you along the way.

Why Set Realistic Goals?

1. Motivation and Focus: Realistic goals provide you with a clear target to work towards, keeping you motivated and focused on your intermittent fasting journey. When you have a specific goal in mind, it becomes easier to stay committed and make the necessary lifestyle changes to achieve it.

2. Sustainability: Setting realistic goals ensures that your intermittent fasting practice is sustainable in the long run. Unrealistic goals, such as aiming for rapid weight loss or extreme fasting durations, can lead to burnout or a sense of failure if they're not achieved. By setting attainable goals, you can maintain a healthy and balanced approach to intermittent fasting.

3. Progress Tracking: Realistic goals allow you to track your progress effectively. When you set achievable milestones, you can measure your success along the way, which provides a sense of accomplishment and encourages you to continue moving forward.

Tips for Setting Realistic Goals

1. Be Specific: Clearly define your goals. Instead of saying, "I want to lose weight," specify how much weight you want to lose and by when. For example, "I want to lose 10 pounds in the

next three months." Specific goals help you stay focused and provide a clear direction.

2. Break It Down: Break your larger goals into smaller, manageable milestones. This helps prevent overwhelm and allows you to celebrate small victories along the way. For instance, if your goal is to fast for 16 hours every day, start by aiming for 12 hours and gradually increase the fasting duration.

3. Consider Your Lifestyle: Take into account your lifestyle, commitments, and personal preferences when setting goals. If you have a busy schedule, it may not be realistic to commit to longer fasting periods every day. Find a balance that works for you and fits seamlessly into your routine.

4. Focus on Non-Scale Victories: While weight loss is a common goal, it's important to focus on other non-scale victories as well. These can include improved energy levels, better sleep quality, increased mental clarity, or improved overall well-being. Acknowledging and celebrating these achievements can keep you motivated and inspired.

5. Be Patient: Rome wasn't built in a day, and neither are sustainable results. Intermittent fasting is a lifestyle change, and it takes time for your body to adapt and for you to see significant changes. Be patient with yourself and trust the process. Remember, slow and steady progress is more sustainable in the long run.

Tracking Your Progress

To track your progress effectively, consider the following

methods:

1. Journaling: Keep a journal to record your fasting hours, meals, and any observations or reflections. This can help you identify patterns, track your progress, and make adjustments as needed.

2. Measurements: In addition to weighing yourself, consider taking body measurements, such as waist circumference, hip circumference, or body fat percentage. These measurements can provide a more comprehensive view of your progress, especially if you're focusing on body composition changes.

3. Photos: Take before and after photos to visually track your progress. Sometimes, changes in your body may not be immediately apparent on the scale, but comparing photos can reveal significant transformations.

4. Well-being Indicators: Pay attention to how you feel overall. Notice changes in energy levels, mood, sleep quality, and other well-being indicators. These subjective measures can be powerful motivators and indicators of progress.

Creating a Fasting Schedule

Creating a fasting schedule is an important step in implementing intermittent fasting into your lifestyle. A well-planned schedule can help you stay consistent, maximize the benefits of fasting, and make it easier to adhere to your chosen fasting method. In this section, we will guide you through the process of creating a fasting schedule that is both engaging and easy to understand.

Understand Your Fasting Method

Before creating a fasting schedule, it's crucial to have a clear understanding of the intermittent fasting method you have chosen. Different methods have varying fasting and eating windows, and it's important to align your schedule accordingly. Whether you're following the 16/8 method, the 5:2 diet, or any other approach, make sure you know the specific guidelines and requirements.

Assess Your Lifestyle and Preferences

When creating a fasting schedule, it's essential to consider your lifestyle and personal preferences. Take into account your work schedule, social commitments, and daily routine. This will help you determine the fasting and eating windows that best fit your lifestyle. For example, if you prefer having breakfast with your family, you may opt for a later eating window.

Determine Your Fasting and Eating Windows

Once you have a clear understanding of your chosen fasting method and have assessed your lifestyle, it's time to determine your fasting and eating windows. Here are some common fasting windows:

1. 16/8 Method: In this method, you fast for 16 hours and have an 8-hour eating window. You can choose the hours that work

best for you. For example, you might fast from 8 pm to 12 pm the next day, and have your meals between 12 pm and 8 pm.

2. 5:2 Diet: With the 5:2 diet, you eat normally for five days of the week and restrict calorie intake to 500-600 calories for the remaining two days. You can choose which days to fast based on your schedule and preferences.

3. Alternate-Day Fasting: Alternate-day fasting involves fasting every other day. On fasting days, you consume little to no calories, while on eating days, you can eat normally. For example, you might fast on Mondays, Wednesdays, and Fridays, and eat normally on the other days.

4. Eat-Stop-Eat: The Eat-Stop-Eat method involves fasting for 24 hours once or twice a week. For example, you might choose to fast from dinner one day until dinner the next day. During the fasting period, only calorie-free beverages are allowed.

5. Warrior Diet: The Warrior Diet follows a 20-hour fasting period, followed by a 4-hour eating window. You can choose the hours that align with your preferences and daily routine.

Plan Your Meals and Snacks

Once you have determined your fasting and eating windows, it's time to plan your meals and snacks accordingly. Ensure that your meals are balanced, nutritious, and aligned with your health goals. Include a variety of whole foods, such as lean proteins, fruits, vegetables, whole grains, and healthy fats. It's also important to stay hydrated throughout the fasting period by consuming water, herbal tea, or other calorie-free beverages.

Adjust and Experiment

Creating a fasting schedule is not a one-size-fits-all approach. It may take some time to find the schedule that works best for you. Be open to adjusting and experimenting with different fasting and eating windows until you find what feels most comfortable and sustainable. Listen to your body and make modifications as needed.

Tips for Success

Here are some additional tips to help you succeed with your fasting schedule:

1. Stay Consistent: Consistency is key when it comes to intermittent fasting. Try to stick to your fasting and eating windows as much as possible to maintain a consistent routine.

2. Be Flexible: While consistency is important, it's also essential to be flexible. Life happens, and there may be occasions when you need to adjust your fasting schedule. Allow yourself the flexibility to adapt without feeling guilty.

3. Stay Hydrated: During the fasting period, it's crucial to stay hydrated. Drink plenty of water and other calorie-free beverages to support your overall well-being.

4. Listen to Your Body: Pay attention to your body's signals and adjust your fasting schedule accordingly. If you feel excessively hungry or fatigued, consider adjusting your fasting window or

seeking guidance from a healthcare professional.

5. Seek Support: Consider joining online communities or finding an accountability partner who is also practicing intermittent fasting. Sharing your experiences, challenges, and successes with others can provide motivation and support along the way.

Creating a fasting schedule is an integral part of incorporating intermittent fasting into your lifestyle. By understanding your chosen method, considering your lifestyle and preferences, and planning your meals accordingly, you can create a schedule that is engaging, easy to understand, and sustainable.

Tips for Successful Intermittent Fasting

Now that you understand the basics, it's time to equip yourself with some practical tips to ensure a successful and enjoyable experience. These tips will help you navigate through the fasting periods, manage hunger and cravings, and optimize your results. Let's dive in!

1. Stay Hydrated

During fasting periods, it's crucial to stay hydrated. Water is your best friend, so make sure to drink an adequate amount throughout the day. Not only will it keep you hydrated, but it can also help curb hunger pangs. Feel free to add a squeeze of lemon or a splash of herbal tea for some flavor variation.

2. Eat Nutrient-Dense Foods

When it's time to break your fast, focus on consuming nutrient-dense foods. Opt for whole, unprocessed foods that are rich in vitamins, minerals, and fiber. Include plenty of fruits, vegetables, lean proteins, and healthy fats in your meals. These foods will provide you with sustained energy and support your overall health.

3. Manage Hunger and Cravings

Hunger and cravings can be challenging during fasting periods, but there are strategies to help you manage them. First, ensure that you're consuming enough calories and nutrients during your eating window to keep you satisfied. Additionally, distractions such as engaging in activities, going for a walk, or practicing mindfulness can help take your mind off food.

4. Incorporate Exercise

Exercise can complement your intermittent fasting journey by boosting your metabolism and promoting fat burning. Aim for a combination of cardiovascular exercises, strength training, and flexibility exercises. However, listen to your body and adjust your exercise routine based on your energy levels during fasting periods.

5. Track Progress and Adjust as Needed

Monitoring your progress is essential to understand how your body responds to intermittent fasting. Keep a journal to track your fasting and eating windows, as well as your food choices and energy levels. Pay attention to how your body feels and make adjustments as needed. Remember, everyone's journey is unique, so find what works best for you.

6. Seek Support and Accountability

Intermittent fasting can be more enjoyable and sustainable when you have support and accountability. Find a friend or join a community of like-minded individuals who are also practicing intermittent fasting. Share your experiences, ask questions, and celebrate your successes together. Having a support system can make a significant difference in your journey.

7. Prioritize Sleep and Stress Management

Sleep and stress play a crucial role in your overall well-being and weight management. Aim for seven to eight hours of quality sleep each night to support your body's natural healing and regeneration processes. Additionally, incorporate stress management techniques such as meditation, deep breathing exercises, or engaging in activities that bring you joy.

8. Be Patient and Flexible

Remember that intermittent fasting is a lifestyle, not a quick fix. Be patient with yourself and your progress. Your body may take time to adjust to the new eating pattern, and weight loss may occur gradually. Embrace the process and be flexible with your fasting and eating windows as needed. Listen to your body and make adjustments accordingly.

By following these tips, you'll set yourself up for success on your intermittent fasting journey. Remember, it's about finding a sustainable and enjoyable approach to eating that works for you. Stay committed, stay positive, and embrace the incredible benefits that intermittent fasting can bring to your life.

Common Myths and Misconceptions about Intermittent Fasting

As intermittent fasting gains popularity, it's important to separate fact from fiction. There are several myths and misconceptions surrounding this eating pattern that can lead to confusion and misinformation. Let's debunk some of the most common myths and set the record straight.

Myth 1: Intermittent Fasting Slows Down Metabolism

One of the most prevalent myths is that intermittent fasting slows down metabolism. However, research suggests that intermittent fasting can actually have a positive impact on metabolic rate. During fasting periods, the body taps into its fat stores for energy, leading to increased fat burning and improved metabolic flexibility.

Myth 2: Intermittent Fasting Leads to Muscle Loss

Many people worry that intermittent fasting will cause muscle loss. However, when done correctly, intermittent fasting can actually help preserve muscle mass. By providing the body with adequate protein and nutrients during the eating window, combined with regular exercise, you can maintain and even build muscle while fasting.

Myth 3: Intermittent Fasting Causes Nutrient Deficiencies

Another common misconception is that intermittent fasting leads to nutrient deficiencies. However, if you focus on consuming a balanced diet rich in whole, nutrient-dense foods during your eating window, you can meet your nutritional needs. It's important to prioritize quality over quantity and ensure that you're getting a variety of vitamins, minerals, and macronutrients.

Myth 4: Intermittent Fasting is Only for Weight Loss

While intermittent fasting can be an effective tool for weight loss, it offers numerous other benefits beyond shedding pounds. Research suggests that intermittent fasting may improve insulin sensitivity, reduce inflammation, support brain health, and promote longevity. It's not just about the numbers on the scale but also about overall health and well-being.

Myth 5: Intermittent Fasting is Not Sustainable

Some people believe that intermittent fasting is not sustainable in the long term. However, many individuals find intermittent fasting to be a sustainable and enjoyable lifestyle. It offers flexibility, allows for social occasions, and can be adapted to fit different schedules and preferences. It's all about finding the approach that works best for you and your lifestyle.

Myth 6: Intermittent Fasting is the Same as Starvation

Intermittent fasting is often misunderstood as starvation, but they are not the same. Starvation is the absence of food for an extended period, leading to severe malnutrition and health complications. Intermittent fasting, on the other hand, involves controlled periods of fasting followed by nourishing meals. It's a structured approach that supports overall health and weight management.

Myth 7: Intermittent Fasting is Only for Certain People

Intermittent fasting is often perceived as suitable only for certain individuals, such as athletes or those with specific health conditions. However, intermittent fasting can be practiced by anyone, as long as they are in good health and have no underlying medical concerns. It's always recommended to consult with a healthcare professional before starting any new dietary regimen.

Myth 8: Intermittent Fasting Requires Skipping Breakfast

Contrary to popular belief, intermittent fasting does not necessarily mean skipping breakfast. While some individuals prefer to skip breakfast and start their eating window later in the day, others may choose to have an early breakfast and finish their eating window earlier. The key is to find a fasting and eating schedule that works best for you and your body.

By debunking these common myths, we can gain a clearer understanding of intermittent fasting and its potential benefits.

Remember, it's important to rely on accurate information and research when making decisions about your health and well-being.

Frequently Asked Questions (FAQ)

<u>What Can I Eat During Intermittent Fasting?</u>

During the fasting period of intermittent fasting, it is recommended to consume only calorie-free beverages such as water, black coffee, or herbal tea. These options will help keep you hydrated and provide some satiety without breaking your fast.

However, during your eating window, you have the freedom to enjoy a variety of foods. It's important to focus on consuming nutrient-dense, whole foods that will nourish your body and support your overall health. Here are some examples of what you can eat during your eating window:

1. Fruits and Vegetables: Include a wide variety of fruits and vegetables in your meals. They are rich in vitamins, minerals, and fiber. Opt for colorful options like berries, leafy greens, broccoli, carrots, and bell peppers.

2. Lean Proteins: Incorporate lean sources of protein such as chicken breast, turkey, fish, tofu, or legumes. Protein is essential for muscle repair and growth.

3. Healthy Fats: Include sources of healthy fats like avocados,

nuts, seeds, olive oil, and coconut oil. These fats provide satiety and support brain health.

4. Whole Grains: If you choose to include grains in your diet, opt for whole grains like quinoa, brown rice, oats, or whole wheat bread. They are higher in fiber and nutrients compared to refined grains.

5. Dairy or Dairy Alternatives: If you tolerate dairy, you can include options like Greek yogurt, cottage cheese, or low-fat milk. If you prefer dairy alternatives, choose unsweetened almond milk, coconut milk, or soy milk.

6. Hydration: Remember to stay hydrated during your eating window as well. Drink plenty of water throughout the day to support your body's functions.

It's important to listen to your body and choose foods that make you feel satisfied and energized. Experiment with different recipes and meal combinations to keep your meals interesting and enjoyable. Remember, intermittent fasting is not about strict dietary restrictions but rather finding a sustainable and balanced approach to eating.

Please note that if you have any specific dietary restrictions or health concerns, it's always best to consult with a healthcare professional or registered dietitian who can provide personalized guidance based on your individual needs.

<u>Can I Drink Coffee or Tea During Fasting?</u>
Absolutely! You can enjoy black coffee or herbal tea during

your fasting period. These beverages are generally considered calorie-free and won't break your fast. However, it's important to avoid adding any sweeteners, milk, cream, or other additives that may contain calories. Stick to plain black coffee or herbal tea for the best results.

Black coffee is a popular choice among intermittent fasters as it can help suppress appetite and provide a boost of energy. Just be mindful of the caffeine content and how it may affect your sleep if consumed later in the day.

Herbal teas, such as chamomile, peppermint, or green tea, are also great options during fasting. They are naturally calorie-free and can provide hydration and a soothing effect.

Remember, the goal of intermittent fasting is to give your body a break from calorie intake, allowing it to tap into stored fat for energy. Coffee and tea can be enjoyed in moderation during the fasting period, but it's important to avoid adding any ingredients that may disrupt the fasting state.

As always, listen to your body and adjust your habits accordingly. If you find that coffee or tea affects your fasting experience negatively, it's best to refrain from consuming them during your fasting window.

How Long Should I Fast for Optimal Results?

The duration of fasting for optimal results can vary depending on individual preferences and goals. There are several popular fasting methods that people follow, each with its own recommended fasting window. Here are a few common fasting methods:

1. 16/8 Method: This method involves fasting for 16 hours and having an 8-hour eating window. It is one of the most popular and beginner-friendly approaches to intermittent fasting. Many people find it manageable to skip breakfast and start their eating window around noon, finishing their last meal of the day by 8 pm.

2. 5:2 Method: With this method, you eat normally for five days of the week and restrict your calorie intake to around 500-600 calories for two non-consecutive days. On fasting days, it's important to focus on nutrient-dense foods to ensure you're getting adequate nutrition.

3. Alternate-Day Fasting: As the name suggests, alternate-day fasting involves fasting every other day. On fasting days, you can consume very few calories (around 500-600) or opt for a complete fast. This method may be more challenging for some individuals, so it's important to listen to your body and adjust as needed.

4. 24-Hour Fast: This method involves fasting for a full 24 hours once or twice a week. For example, you may choose to fast from dinner one day until dinner the next day. It's important to stay hydrated during this fasting period and break your fast with a balanced meal.

The optimal fasting duration may vary depending on factors such as individual goals, lifestyle, and overall health. It's important to choose a fasting method that feels sustainable and fits well with your routine. It's also crucial to prioritize nutrient-dense foods during your eating window to ensure you're meeting your nutritional needs.

If you're new to intermittent fasting, it's recommended to start with a shorter fasting window, such as the 16/8 method, and gradually increase the duration as you become more comfortable.

Remember, consistency is key when it comes to intermittent fasting. Find a fasting schedule that works for you and stick to it. It's also important to listen to your body and make adjustments if needed. If you have any underlying health conditions or concerns, it's always best to consult with a healthcare professional before starting any new dietary regimen.

Is Intermittent Fasting Safe for Everyone?

Intermittent fasting can be safe for many individuals, but it may not be suitable for everyone. It's important to consider your individual health status, medical conditions, and any medications you may be taking before starting an intermittent fasting regimen. It's always recommended to consult with a healthcare professional or registered dietitian before making any significant changes to your diet or lifestyle.

While intermittent fasting has been shown to have various health benefits, it may not be appropriate for individuals who:

1. Have a history of disordered eating: Intermittent fasting may trigger or worsen disordered eating patterns in individuals with a history of eating disorders. It's important to prioritize

a healthy relationship with food and seek guidance from a healthcare professional if you have a history of disordered eating.

2. Are pregnant or breastfeeding: Pregnancy and lactation are times when adequate nutrition is crucial for both the mother and the baby. Intermittent fasting may not provide sufficient nutrients during these periods, so it's best to focus on a balanced diet recommended by healthcare professionals.

3. Have certain medical conditions: Individuals with certain medical conditions, such as diabetes, low blood sugar (hypoglycemia), or a history of gastric ulcers, may need to approach intermittent fasting with caution or avoid it altogether. It's important to consult with a healthcare professional who can provide personalized guidance based on your specific condition.

4. Take certain medications: Some medications may require regular food intake or may interact with fasting. If you take medications, it's important to consult with your healthcare professional to ensure that intermittent fasting will not interfere with their effectiveness or safety.

5. Are underweight or have a history of nutrient deficiencies: Intermittent fasting may not be suitable for individuals who are underweight or have a history of nutrient deficiencies. It's important to prioritize adequate nutrition and consult with a healthcare professional to ensure that your nutritional needs are being met.

Remember, the safety and suitability of intermittent fasting can vary from person to person. It's crucial to prioritize your health and well-being above all else. Consulting with a healthcare professional or registered dietitian will help you determine if intermittent fasting is appropriate for you and how to approach it in a safe and sustainable manner.

<u>Can I Exercise While Fasting?</u>

Certainly! Exercising while fasting is generally safe and can even have some benefits. However, it's important to listen to your body and make adjustments as needed. Here are some considerations for exercising during fasting:

1. Timing: If you're following the 16/8 method of intermittent fasting, you may choose to exercise towards the end of your fasting period, right before breaking your fast. This way, you can replenish your energy stores with a post-workout meal. However, if you prefer to exercise during your eating window, that is also perfectly fine.

2. Hydration: Staying hydrated is crucial, especially when exercising. Make sure to drink plenty of water before, during, and after your workout to maintain proper hydration levels.

3. Intensity: If you're new to fasting or exercise, it's important to start slowly and gradually increase the intensity of your workouts. Pay attention to how your body responds and adjust accordingly. If you feel lightheaded, dizzy, or excessively fatigued, it may be a sign to dial back the intensity or consider breaking your fast before exercising.

4. Fueling: If you're planning a more intense or prolonged workout, you may benefit from consuming a small pre-workout snack that includes a combination of carbohydrates and protein. This can help provide some energy and support muscle recovery. Opt for easily digestible options such as a banana with nut butter or a small protein shake.

5. Post-workout meal: After your workout, it's important to refuel your body with a balanced meal that includes protein, carbohydrates, and healthy fats. This will help replenish glycogen stores, support muscle repair, and aid in recovery.

Remember, everyone's body is different, and what works for one person may not work for another. It's important to listen to your body, make adjustments as needed, and prioritize your overall well-being. If you have any specific health concerns or medical conditions, it's always best to consult with a healthcare professional or registered dietitian before starting an exercise routine while fasting.

Conclusion

Intermittent fasting is a popular dietary approach that involves cycling between periods of fasting and eating. It has gained significant attention for its potential health benefits and effectiveness in weight management. Throughout this book, we have explored the concept of intermittent fasting, its various methods, and its impact on our bodies.

Intermittent fasting offers more than just a way to shed a few pounds. It has been shown to have positive effects on insulin sensitivity, cellular repair processes, and even brain health. By giving our bodies a break from constant calorie intake, we allow it to tap into stored fat for energy, leading to potential weight loss and improved metabolic health.

However, it's important to note that intermittent fasting may not be suitable for everyone. Individuals with certain medical conditions, a history of disordered eating, or who are pregnant or breastfeeding should exercise caution and consult with a healthcare professional before starting an intermittent fasting regimen.

When embarking on an intermittent fasting journey, it's crucial to choose a fasting method that aligns with your lifestyle and goals. Whether it's the 16/8 method, the 5:2 approach, or alternate-day fasting, finding a schedule that works for you is key to long-term success.

To optimize your intermittent fasting experience, consider incorporating nutrient-dense foods into your eating window. Focus on whole grains, lean proteins, fruits, vegetables, and healthy fats to ensure you're meeting your nutritional needs.

Additionally, staying hydrated, getting regular exercise, and prioritizing quality sleep are important factors to support your overall health and well-being while fasting.

Remember, intermittent fasting is not a quick fix or a one-size-fits-all solution. It requires commitment, patience, and an understanding of your body's needs. It's essential to listen to your body, make adjustments as necessary, and seek guidance from healthcare professionals or registered dietitians if needed.

Incorporating intermittent fasting into your lifestyle can be a powerful tool for improving your health and achieving your wellness goals. However, it's important to approach it with a balanced mindset and a focus on overall well-being.

So, if you're considering intermittent fasting, take the time to educate yourself, consult with professionals, and embark on this journey with confidence. Remember, it's not just about the weight loss, but also about embracing a healthier lifestyle and nurturing your body from within.

Now, armed with the knowledge and understanding of intermittent fasting, you can make informed decisions about whether it's the right approach for you. So, go ahead, explore the possibilities, and may your intermittent fasting journey be filled with health, vitality, and success!

Thanks

Thank you, dear reader, for embarking on this journey through the world of intermittent fasting with us. We hope that this book has provided you with valuable insights and knowledge to make informed decisions about incorporating intermittent fasting into your lifestyle.

If you found this book helpful and enjoyable, we would greatly appreciate it if you could take a moment to leave a review. Your feedback is invaluable to us and helps us continue to create content that resonates with our readers.

Furthermore, if you know someone who might benefit from learning about intermittent fasting, we encourage you to share this book with them. Together, we can spread the knowledge and empower others to make positive changes in their health and well-being.

Wishing you health, vitality, and success on your intermittent fasting journey!